CARNIVORE DIET COOKBOOK FOR WOMEN

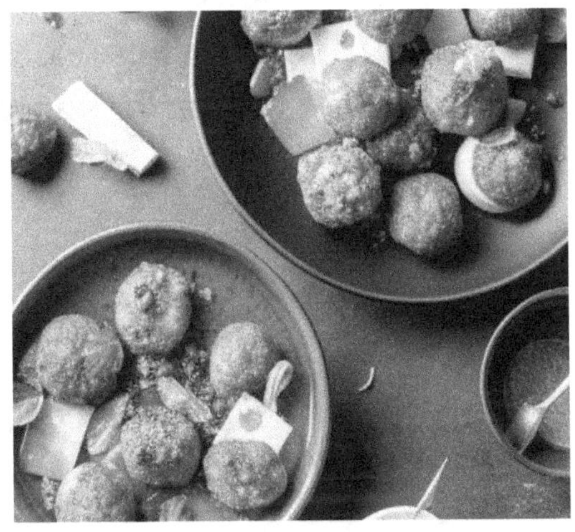

Easy and Delicious Recipes for Carnivore Dieters

JESSICA MURRAY

Copyright © 2023 Jessica Murray

All Rights Reserved. No part of this book may be reproduced in any form or by any electronic or mechanical means, including information storage and retrieval systems, without written permission from the publisher, except for the inclusion of brief quotations in a review.

Dear Reader,

Thank you for the purchase. I hope you enjoy and love it, would you consider dropping an honest feedback/review, I will appreciate that and you can contact me using JessicaMurrayDietHelp@gmail.com if you have any questions, I will gladly respond

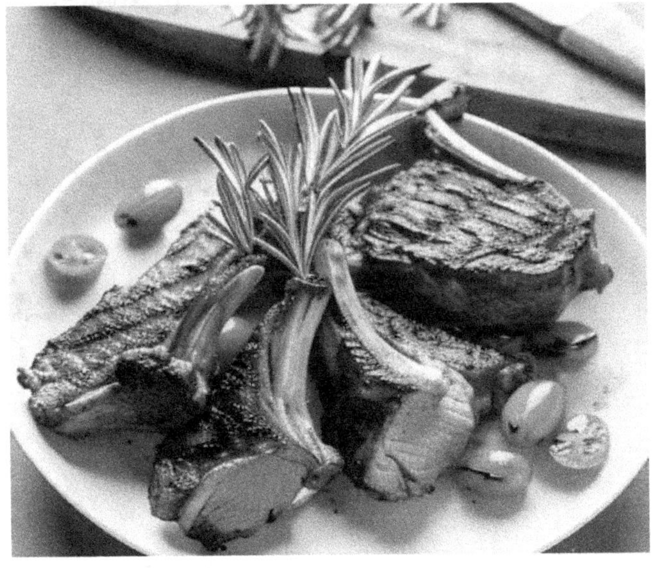

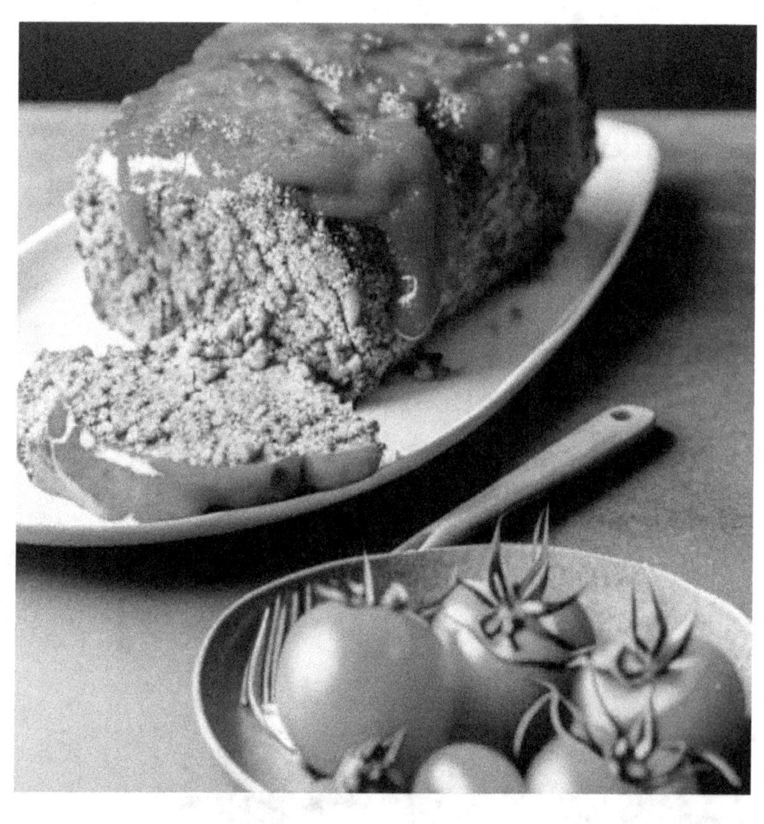

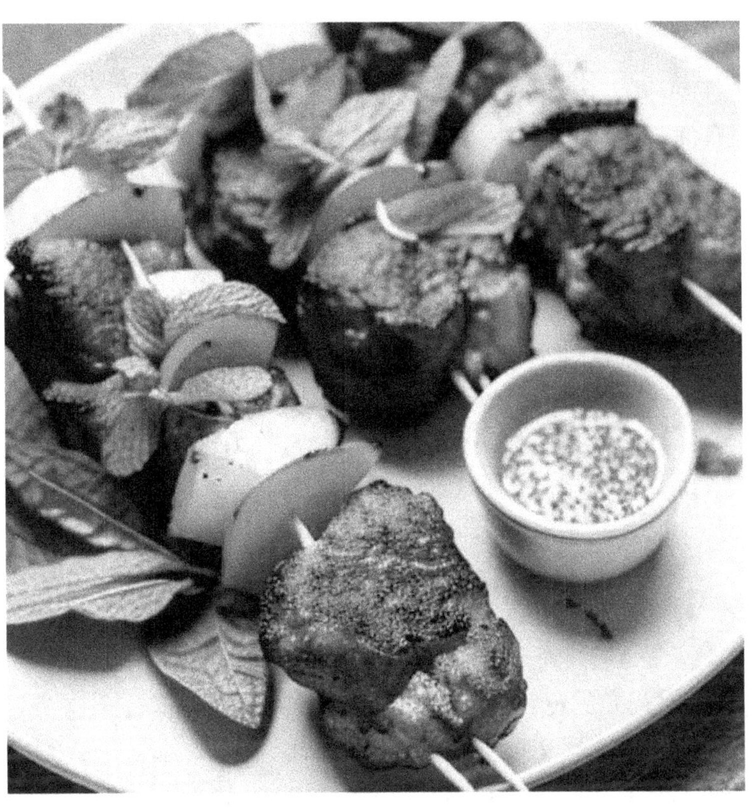

Table of Contents

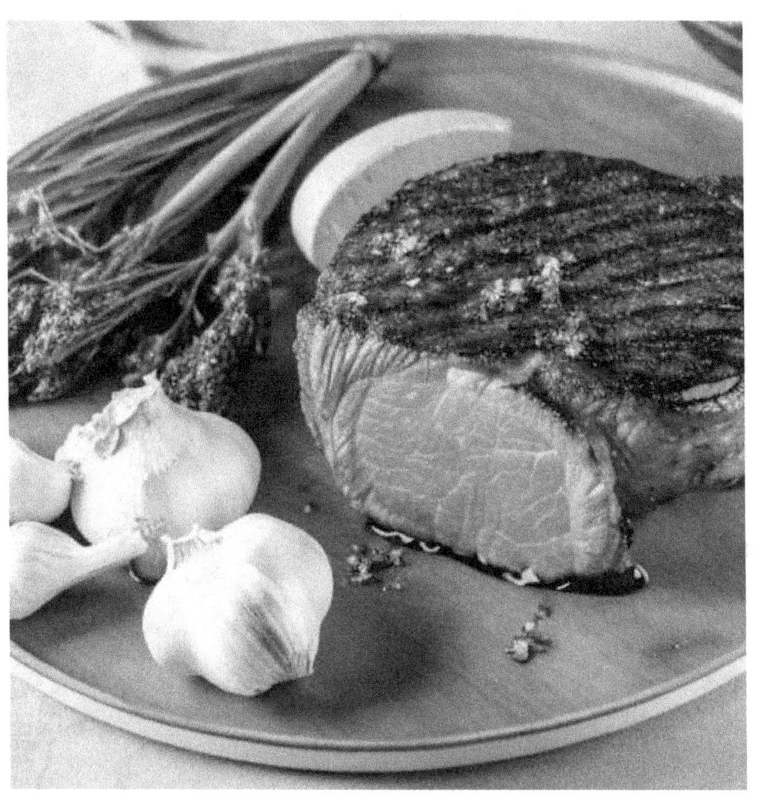

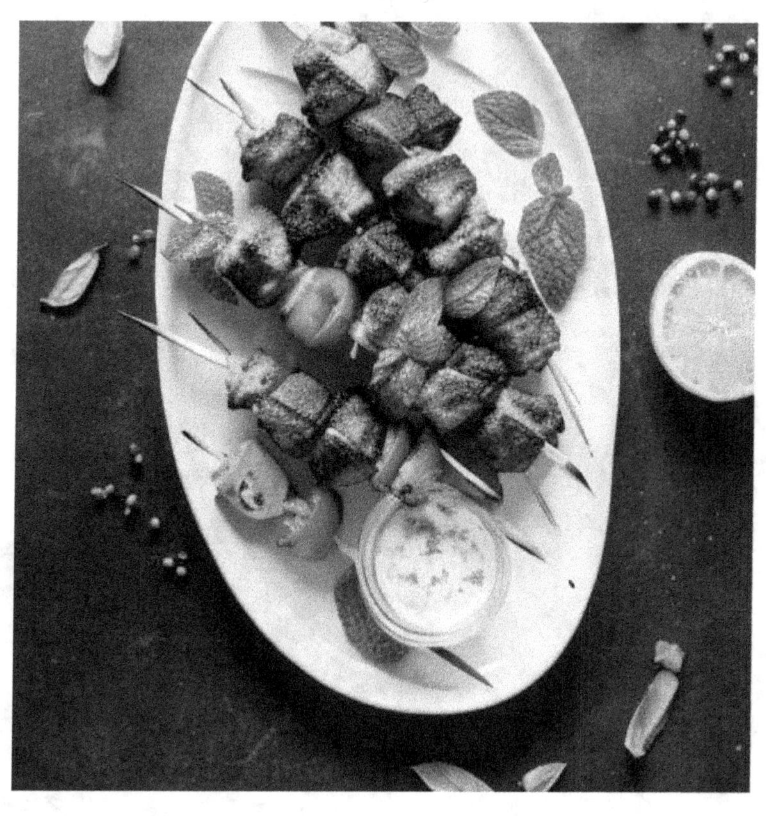

INTRODUCTION TO THE CARNIVORE DIET FOR WOMEN

For years, Beth had been having difficulty losing weight. She attempted numerous diets to no avail. Suddenly, one day she heard about the Carnivore Diet specifically designed for women. Initially, she was uncertain, but she decided to give it a chance. After only two weeks, she noticed changes in her body. She felt more energetic and no longer had cravings for junk food. She stayed on the diet and after six months, she had lost a remarkable 15 pounds! She was astounded by the results and was so thankful she tried the Carnivore Diet created for women.

Benefits of the Carnivore Diet for Women

1. Better Hormonal Balance: The carnivore diet's high-protein, low-carb diet promotes hormone balance, which may be particularly advantageous for women.

2. Increased Energy: The body receives a consistent flow of energy from solely eating animal proteins and lipids, which helps to reduce weariness and increase alertness.

3. Better Gut Health: The carnivore diet's high fat content helps to lower gut inflammation, which can enhance digestion and nutrient absorption.

4. Lessened Cravings: The carnivore diet helps to lessen cravings for harmful foods by cutting out processed and sugary foods, enabling better control over eating patterns.

5. Weight loss: The carnivore diet can help with weight loss because it is heavy in protein and fat and low in carbs.

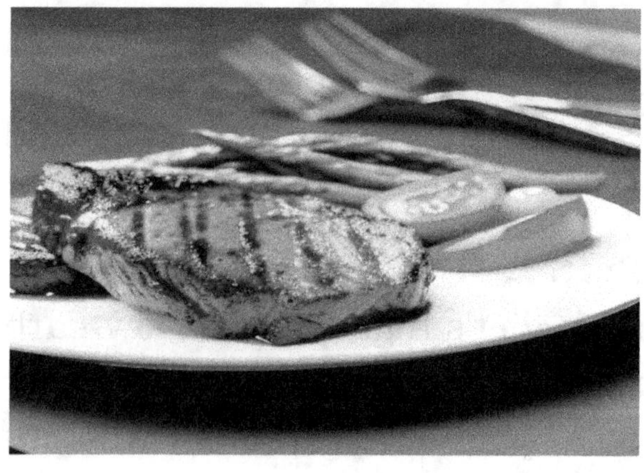

CHAPTER 1

BREAKFAST RECIPES

Fried Eggs and Bacon

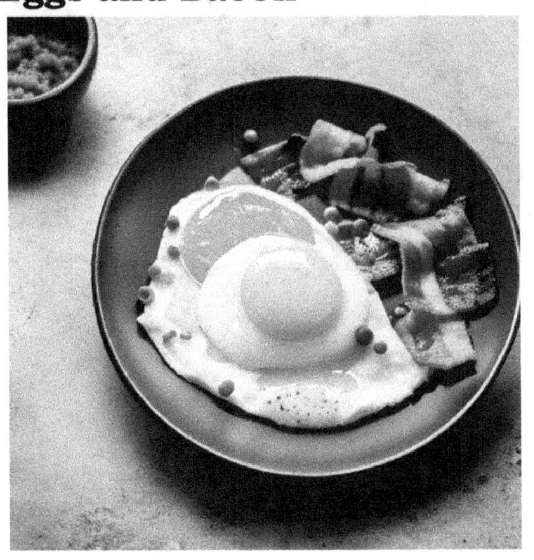

Ingredients:

- 2 eggs, 3-5 pieces of bacon

Instructions:

- • Set a skillet over medium heat. Add the bacon pieces and fry until crisp once heated.
- Place the bacon on a platter and leave it there. Into the same skillet, crack eggs. Fry eggs until desired doneness is reached.

- Serve bacon and eggs.

Grilled Steak and Eggs

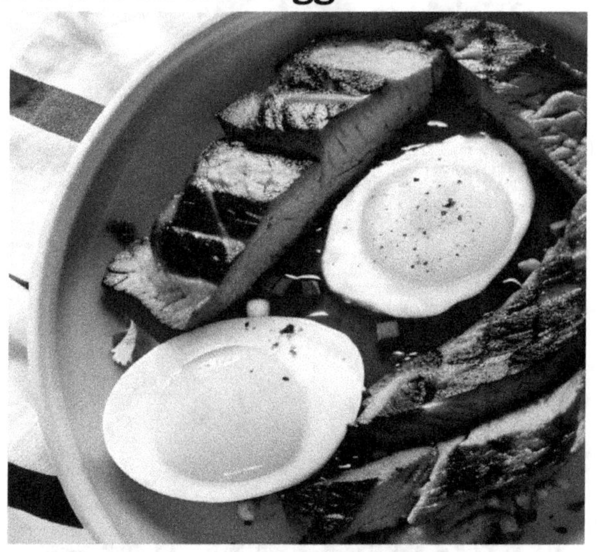

Ingredients:
- 4-6 oz. steak, 2-3 eggs

Instructions:
- A pan or griddle should be heated to medium-high heat.
- Add preferred spices and seasonings to the steak. For medium-rare, place the steak on the griddle or in a pan and cook for about 4 minutes on each side.

- Steak should be removed and rested for five minutes. In the same skillet, lower the heat to medium-low and add the eggs.
- Fry eggs until they are the desired doneness. Serve the eggs and steak together.

Ribeye Steak with Garlic Butter

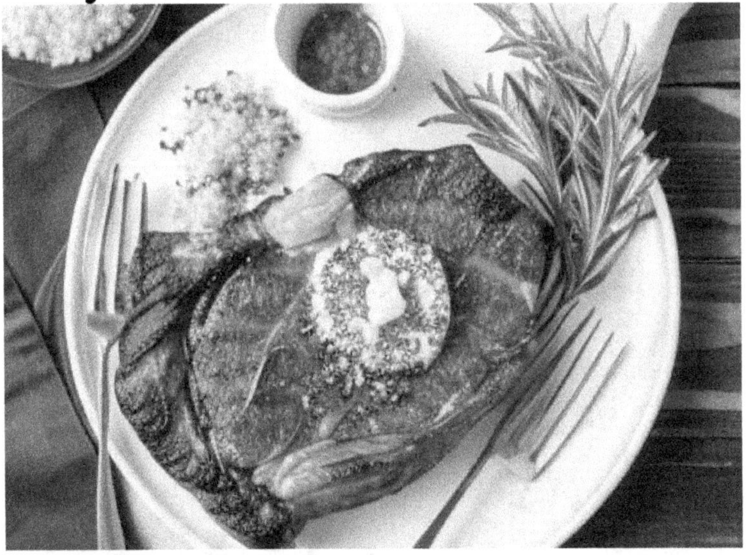

Ingredients:
- 2 steaks, ribeye
- 4 tsp. unsalted butter
- 2 minced garlic cloves
- 2 teaspoons minced fresh parsley
- Taste-tested salt and pepper

Instructions:

- Set the oven to 375 degrees.
- Place each steak on a baking pan after seasoning with salt and pepper.
- Gently heat the butter in a small pot.
- Stirring constantly, sauté the garlic and parsley for 2 minutes.
- Liberally apply the garlic butter to each steak.
- Bake the steaks in the preheated oven for 10 to 15 minutes, depending on the desired degree of doneness.

Bacon and beef burgers

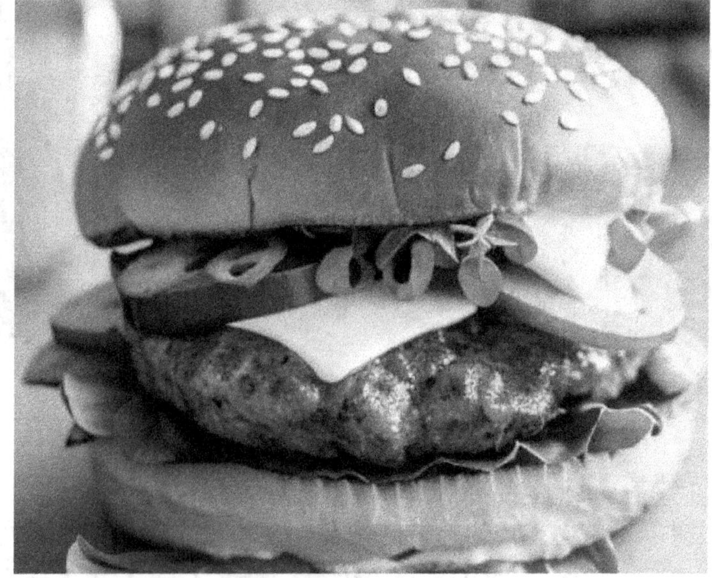

Ingredients:

- 1 pound of beef.

- Four pieces of chopped and cooked bacon.
- 1/2 cup chopped onions
- 1 minced garlic clove
- 1/4 cup of breadcrumbs
- 1 lightly beaten egg
- Worcestershire sauce, two tablespoons
- Taste-tested salt and pepper

Instructions:

- Combine the bread crumbs, egg, Worcestershire sauce, salt, and pepper in a big bowl with the ground beef, bacon, onions, garlic, and bread crumbs.
- Create 4 patties out of the mixture.
- Preheat a large skillet over medium heat, add the patties, and cook for 12 minutes, rotating once halfway through, or until thoroughly cooked.

Lamb Chops with Rosemary

Ingredients:

- 4 chops of lamb
- Olive oil, two tablespoons
- 1 teaspoon minced fresh rosemary
- 2 minced garlic cloves
- Taste-tested salt and pepper

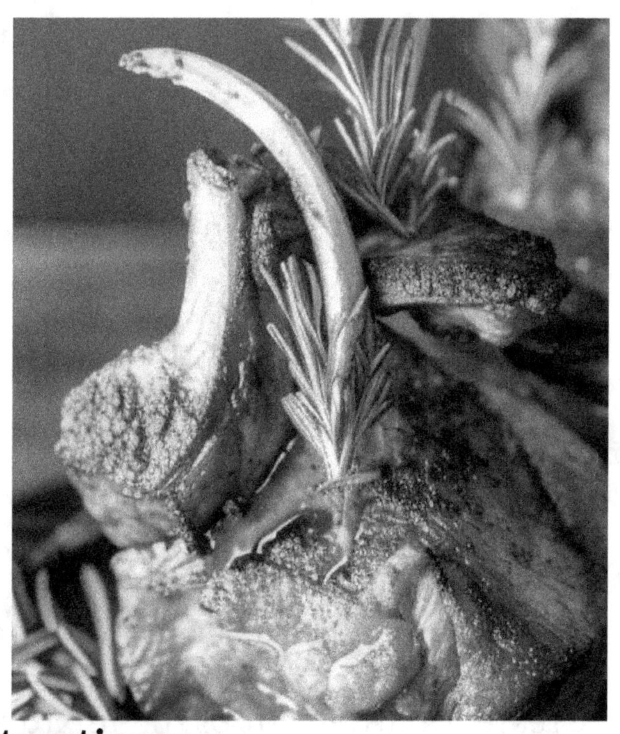

Instructions:

- Set the oven to 375 degrees.
- Season the lamb chops with salt, pepper, rosemary, garlic, and olive oil.
- Arrange the lamb chops on a baking sheet and bake for 15 minutes, or until desired doneness is reached, in a preheated oven.

Venison Meatloaf with Tomato Glaze

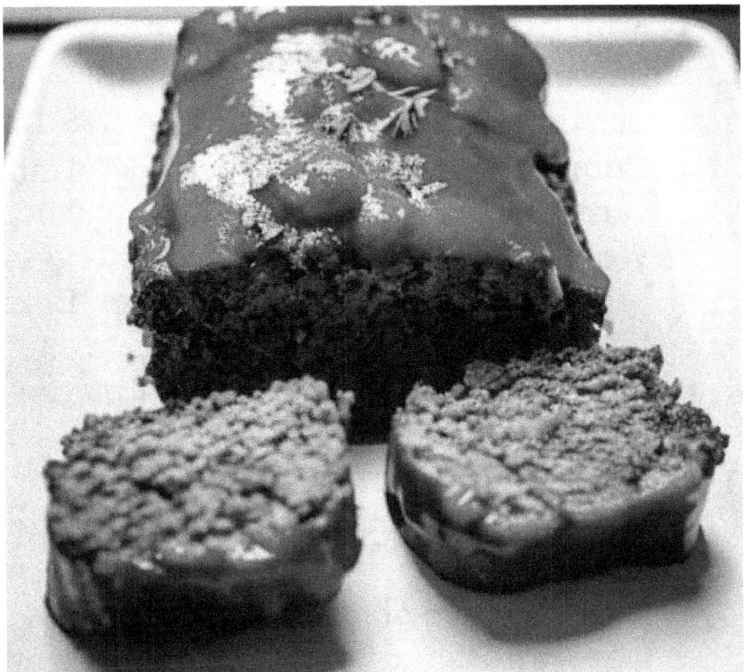

Ingredients:

- 1 lb. each of ground venison and beef,
- 1/2 diced onion, 2 minced garlic cloves,
- 1 tbs. of Worcestershire sauce, 2 beaten eggs,
- 1/2 cup of breadcrumbs, salt, and pepper, as well as 1/2 cup of ketchup,
- 2 tbs. of brown sugar,

- 1 tbs. of Worcestershire sauce,
- and 1 tsp. of dried oregano

Instructions:

- Set the oven's temperature to 375 F.
- Combine the ground beef, ground venison, onion, garlic, Worcestershire sauce, eggs, breadcrumbs, salt, and pepper in a big bowl.
- Shape into a loaf and set in a baking dish that has been buttered.
- Combine the ketchup, brown sugar, Worcestershire sauce, and oregano in a small bowl.
- Cover the top of the meatloaf with the glaze and bake for 45 to 1 hour, or until the middle is well cooked.
- Wait 10 minutes before serving the meatloaf to let it cool.

CHAPTER 2

LUNCH RECIPES

Bison Chili

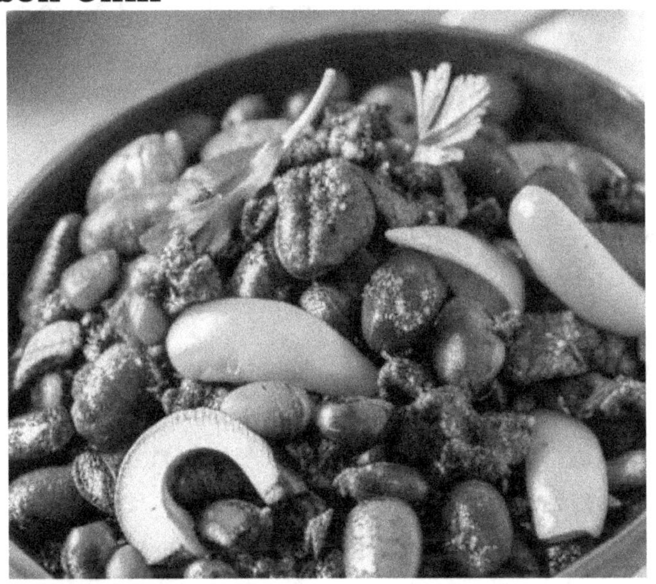

Ingredients:

- Olive oil, two tablespoons
- 1 sliced onion
- 2 minced garlic cloves
- 1 pound of ground bison
- One (14.5 ounce) can of diced tomatoes.
- One can (4 Oz) of green Chiles
- Two teaspoons of chili powder
- 1/2 tsp. cumin
- 1/2 tsp. oregano

- 1/2 tsp. paprika
- 1/4 teaspoon cayenne
- Taste-tested salt and pepper
- 1 (15 Oz) can rinsed and drained black beans

Instructions:

- In a big pot over medium heat, warm the olive oil.
- Stir in the onion and garlic, cooking for a further 2 minutes or until softened.
- The heat is raised to medium-high, and the ground beef is added. Cook while stirring occasionally until browned.
- Lower the heat to medium-low and add the chopped tomatoes, green Chiles, cumin, paprika, cayenne pepper, salt, and pepper. Also add chili powder, oregano, and paprika. To blend, stir.
- Simmer until thickened, about 10-15 minutes.
- Add the black beans and cook for an additional 5 minutes, or until thoroughly cooked.

Chicken Liver Pate
Ingredients:
- 1 pound of chicken livers
- 1 sliced onion
- 2 minced garlic cloves
- Four teaspoons of butter
- White wine, 1/4 cup
- 2 teaspoons minced fresh parsley
- Brandy, two teaspoons
- Worcestershire sauce, two tablespoons
- Taste-tested salt and pepper

Instructions:
- Ina a skillet with a large surface area and medium temperature, the butter is melted
- Stir in the onion and garlic, cooking for a further 3 minutes or until softened.
- The heat is raised to medium-high, and the chicken livers are added. Cook until browned, about 4–5 minutes.
- Lower the heat to a low setting and stir in the brandy, white wine, parsley, Worcestershire sauce, salt, and pepper. 3 minutes of simmering.

- Spoon the mixture into a food processor, and run the machine until it's smooth.

Turkey Burger with Avocado

Ingredients:

- 1pound ground turkey,
- Half a teaspoon of each of the following: garlic powder, onion powder, salt, and pepper,
- 1/4 cup BBQ sauce, 1 avocado, sliced, 4 hamburger buns,
- 1/4 cup shredded cheddar cheese

Instructions:

- Preheat a grill to medium-high heat.
- In a medium bowl, combine the ground turkey, garlic powder, onion powder, salt, and pepper. Mix until evenly combined.
- Form the ground turkey into 4 patties.
- Grill the patties for 5 minutes on each side.
- Cook the patties for a further five minutes after flipping.
- Brush each patty with BBQ sauce.

- Place the patties on the buns and top with avocado slices and shredded cheese.
- Serve.

Beef and Broccoli Stir Fry

Ingredients:

- 1pound flank steak, 1 tablespoon olive oil, 2 cloves garlic, minced,
- 2 cups broccoli florets, 1/2 cup low sodium beef broth
- 1/4 cup soy sauce, 1 tablespoon cornstarch,
- 2 teaspoons sesame oil, 1 teaspoon sugar, Salt and pepper to taste

Instructions:

- Cut the steak into thin strips.
- Heat the olive oil in a large skillet over medium-high heat.
- Stir-fry the garlic for one minute after adding it.
- Stir-fry the steak strips for 3–4 minutes after adding them.
- Add the broccoli and stir-fry for an additional 3-4 minutes.

- In a small bowl, combine the beef broth, soy sauce, cornstarch, sesame oil, sugar, and salt and pepper. Whisk until combined.
- Pour the mixture into the skillet and cook for 2-3 minutes, or until the sauce thickens.
- Serve.

Bacon Lettuce Tomato Salad
Ingredients:
- 4 slices of bacon, cooked and crumbled,
- 4 cups romaine lettuce, chopped,
- 1/2 cup cherry tomatoes, halved,
- 1/4 cup red onion, diced,
- 2 tablespoons olive oil, 1 tablespoon red wine vinegar,
- 1/2 teaspoon Dijon mustard, Salt and pepper to taste

Instructions:
- In a large bowl, combine the romaine lettuce, cherry tomatoes, red onion, and bacon.

- Combine the olive oil, red wine vinegar, Dijon mustard, salt, and pepper in a small bowl.
- Drizzle the salad with the dressing, then toss to incorporate.
- Serve.

Keto-Friendly Beef Jerky
Ingredients:

- 2 pounds of beef (any cut) cut into thin strips
- 1/2 cup sugar-free teriyaki sauce
- 2 teaspoons of smoked paprika
- 1 teaspoon each of garlic powder, onion powder, and pepper, and
- 1/2 teaspoon of crushed black pepper.

Instructions:

- Set the oven's temperature to 175 degrees.
- blend the teriyaki sauce, smoked paprika, garlic powder, onion powder, and ground black pepper in a sizable bowl and stir to blend.
- Add the beef strips to the marinade, making sure to completely cover each piece.

- Arrange the beef strips on a baking sheet that has been buttered, making sure they don't touch.
- Bake for 3 to 4 hours at 175 degrees Fahrenheit to achieve the required jerky consistency.
- Prior to plating for consumption, allow the dish to cool down for a period of 15 minutes.

DINNER RECIPES

Grilled Beef Steak

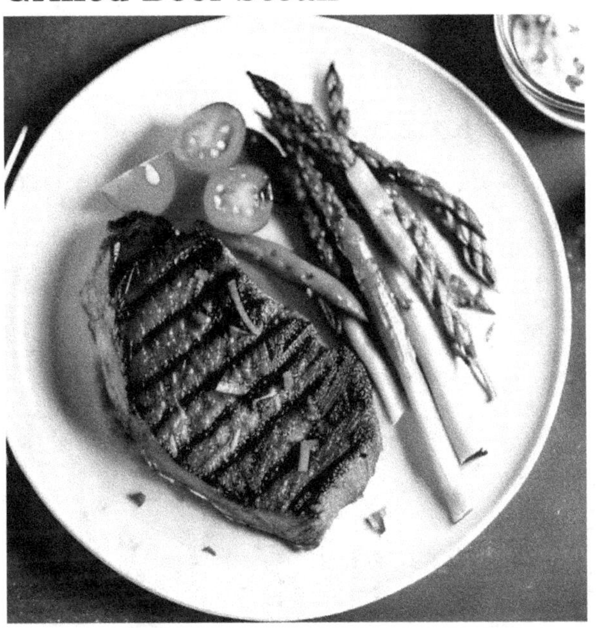

Ingredients:

- two to three pounds of beef steak, one teaspoon of coarse salt, one teaspoon of ground black pepper,
- one tablespoon of vegetable oil, and one tablespoon of garlic powder.

Instructions:

- Turn the grill's heat up to medium-high.

- Sprinkle salt, pepper, garlic powder, and vegetable oil on the meat.
- Grill the steak for about 7 minutes on each side, or until it is cooked to your liking.
- After taking the steak from the grill, let it five minutes to rest before serving.

Beef Liver with Onions and Bacon

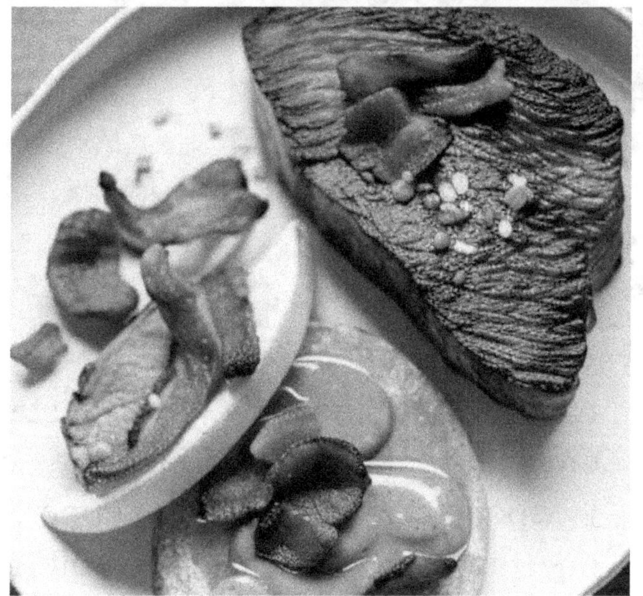

Ingredients:

- 1 pound of beef liver, diced into 1-inch-long chunks
- 4 chopped pieces of bacon

- 1 sliced onion
- 2 minced garlic cloves
- 1/2 cup beef stock
- 2 teaspoons minced fresh parsley
- Taste-tested salt and pepper

Instructions:

- Turn on the medium-high heat under a sizable skillet.
- Add the bacon and heat, stirring periodically, until crispy.
- Using a slotted spoon, remove the bacon, leaving the produced fat in the skillet.
- Add the onion and garlic and simmer for a few minutes until soft.
- Include the beef liver and simmer for a further 4-5 minutes, or until browned.
- Include the bacon, parsley, beef broth, salt, and pepper. Simmer the liquid for 5 minutes, or until it has reduced.

Bacon-Wrapped Asparagus

Ingredients:

- 1 pound of asparagus spears,
- 4 to 5 pieces of bacon,

- 2 tablespoons extra virgin olive oil, salt, and black pepper

Instructions:

- Set the oven's temperature to 400 degrees.
- Combine the asparagus spears, extra virgin olive oil, salt, and pepper in a big bowl.
- Divide the bacon slices into thirds and around each asparagus spear with a piece.
- Arrange the asparagus spears with bacon wrappers on a prepared baking sheet.
- Bake the bacon for 15 to 20 minutes at 400 degrees Fahrenheit to make it crispy.
- Remove the dish from the inside of the oven.

Lamb Kebabs with Mint Yogurt Sauce

Ingredients:

- 1 lb. minced lamb
- 1 finely chopped onion,
- 1/2 cup chopped fresh mint leaves,
- 1 tbs. olive oil, 1/2 cup plain Greek yogurt, and
- 1 tbs. freshly squeezed lemon juice.

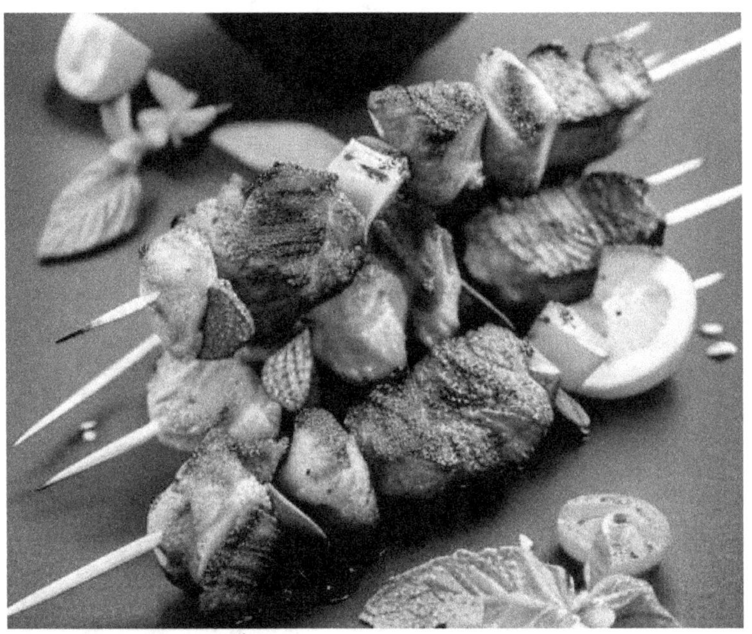

Instructions:

- Set the heat of the grill to a medium-to-high level.
- Combine ground lamb, onion, mint, cumin, garlic powder, and coarsely powdered black pepper in a big bowl.
- Create 8 to 10 tiny kebabs out of the ingredients.
- Apply olive oil to the kebabs on both sides.
- When the kebabs are done, flip them over at least once. Grill them for 10 to 12 minutes.

- In a separate bowl, combine the Greek yogurt, lemon juice, salt, and pepper to make the yogurt sauce.
- Spoon the yogurt sauce over the kebabs.

Cumin-Spiced Beef Ribs

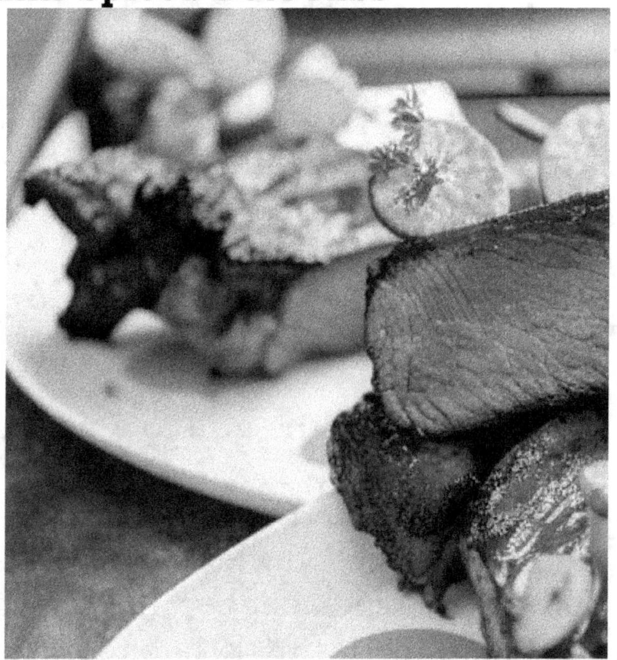

Ingredients:

- 4-5 pounds of beef ribs,
- 2 tablespoons of smoked paprika,
- 2 tablespoons of ground cumin,
- 2 tablespoons of garlic powder,
- 1 tablespoon of onion powder,
- 1 tablespoon of dried oregano,

- 2 tablespoons of Worcestershire sauce,
- 2 tablespoons of olive oil, salt, and black pepper.

Instructions:
- Turn the oven's temperature up to 350 degrees.
- Combine smoked paprika, cumin, oregano, brown sugar, Worcestershire sauce, and olive oil in a mixture and rub it on the ribs.
- Sprinkle salt and black pepper on the ribs.
- Put the ribs in a roasting pan and wrap them in foil.
- Roast the ribs for 2.5 to 3 hours in the oven, or until they are fork-tender.
- Take the ribs out of the oven and dish them out.

Grilled Swordfish Steaks

Ingredients:
- 6-8 Ounce swordfish steaks,
- 2 tablespoons of olive oil,
- 2 minced garlic cloves,
- 2 tablespoons of freshly squeezed lemon juice,

- 2 tablespoons of chopped fresh parsley, salt, and black pepper.

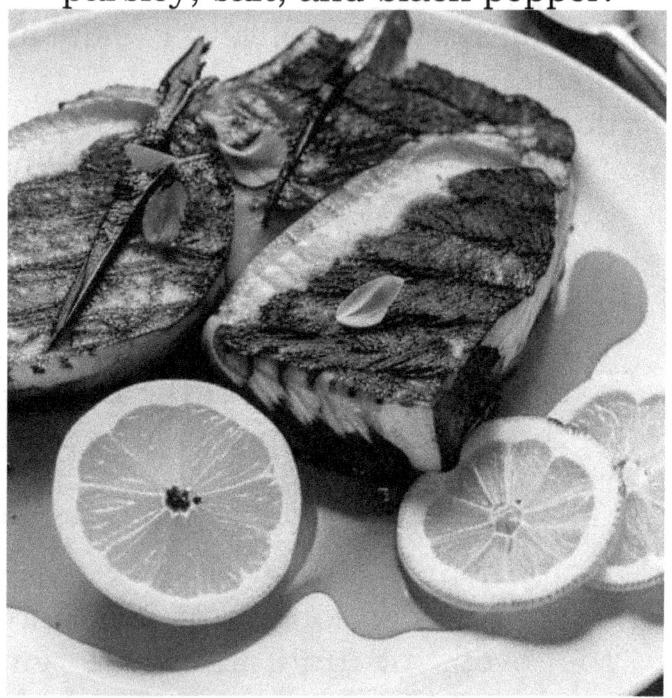

Instructions:

- The heat of the grill should be adjusted to a level that is somewhere in the range of medium to high.
- Combine the olive oil, garlic, lemon juice, parsley, salt, and pepper in a sizable bowl.
- Apply the marinade with a brush to the swordfish steaks.

- Grill the swordfish for 5 to 7 minutes on each side, or until it is thoroughly cooked.
- Move to a plate and offer.

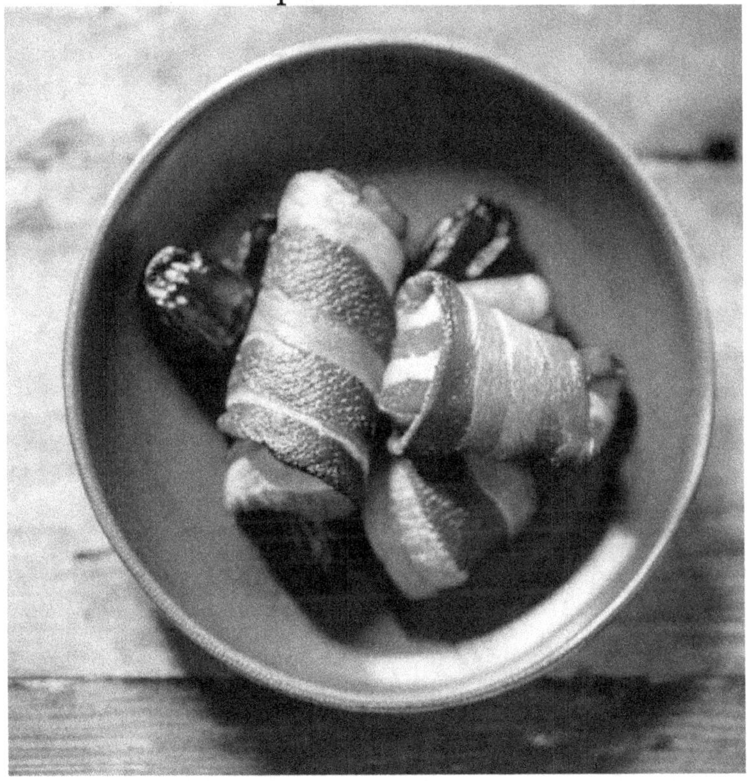

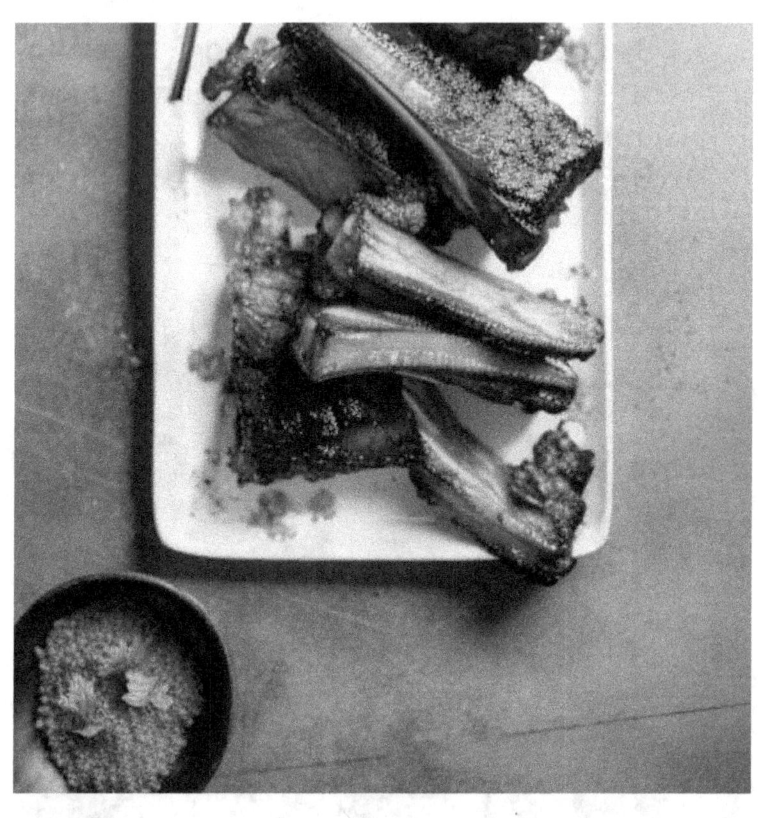

CHAPTER 4

SNACKS AND DESSERTS

Bacon-Wrapped Dates

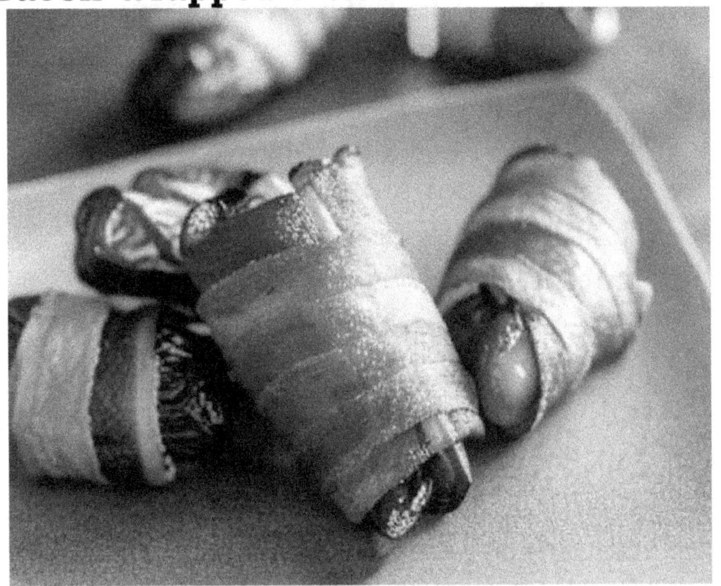

Ingredients:
- 12 large medjool dates
- and 12 pieces of bacon.

Instructions:
- Set the oven to 375 degrees.
- Halve each bacon slice, then wrap one half around each date.
- Arrange the dates on a foil-lined baking pan.

* Bake for about 20 minutes in a preheated oven, or until bacon is crisp.

Grilled Pineapple with Prosciutto

Ingredients

* 1 large pineapple, peeled, cored, and sliced
* 2 tablespoons olive oil –
* 12 slices of prosciutto

Instructions:

* Set a grill outside to medium-high heat.
* Olive oil should be brushed over the pineapple segments.
* Grill the pineapple slices for about 3 minutes, or until they are just beginning to brown.
* After turning the pineapple over, add a slice of prosciutto to each piece, and cook for an additional 3 minutes, or until the prosciutto is crisp and cooked through.

Beef Jerky Bites

Ingredients:

* 2 pounds of thinly sliced beef top round and 1/4 cup soy sauce.

- One-fourth cup of Worcestershire sauce
- 1 teaspoon of garlic powder
- 2 teaspoons of honey
- One tablespoon of onion powder
- one teaspoon of smoked paprika

Instructions:
- Turn the oven on to 175F.
- Put the meat cutlets in a big bowl.
- Combine the soy sauce, Worcestershire sauce, honey, garlic powder, onion powder, and smoked paprika in a separate bowl.
- Add the meat slices to the mixture and toss to coat.
- Arrange the beef slices on a parchment-lined baking sheet and bake for 3 to 5 hours, depending on the texture you want, in the preheated oven.

Deviled Eggs with Bacon Crumbles
Ingredients:
- 6 big eggs
- 1/8 cup mayonnaise
- One tablespoon of Dijon mustard
- To taste, salt and pepper

- 2 cooked and crumbled slices of bacon

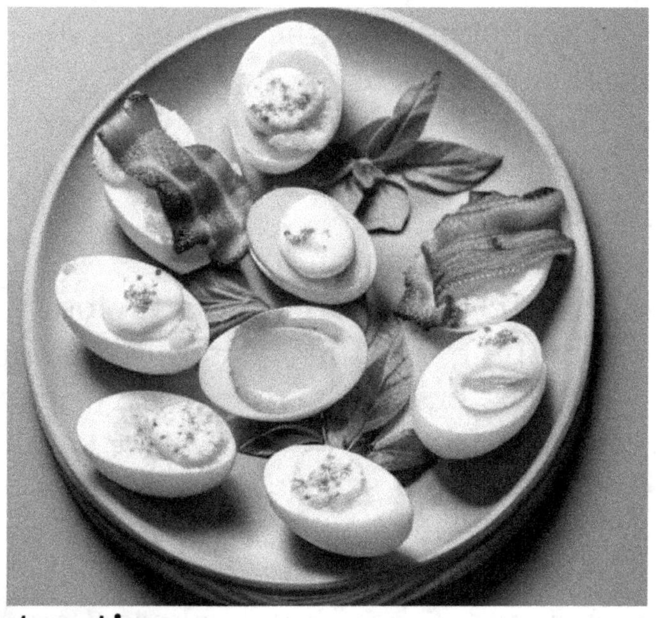

Instructions:

- Put the eggs in a medium saucepan and cover with cold water so that the water is 1 inch over the eggs.
- Use a medium-high heat source to bring the water to a boil.
- After the water has reached a rolling boil, turn the heat down to low, cover the pan, and simmer the eggs for 12 minutes.
- Move the eggs to an ice bath, where they should chill for five minutes.

- After removing the eggs' shells, cut them in half lengthwise.
- Take out the yolks and put them in a little basin.
- Stir the mayonnaise, Dijon mustard, salt, and pepper into the yolks after mashing them with a fork.
- Add some bacon crumbles on top after spooning the yolk mixture into the egg halves.

Sausage Stuffed Mushrooms

Ingredients:
- 12 large button mushrooms
- 1/4 cup breadcrumbs
- 1/2 Pound ground sausage
- 1/4 cup Parmesan cheese, grated - 2 minced garlic cloves
- 2 teaspoons freshly chopped parsley
- To taste, salt and pepper

Instructions:
- Set the oven to 375 degrees.
- Cut the mushroom stems off and set them aside.
- Combine the sausage, breadcrumbs, Parmesan cheese, garlic, parsley, and salt and pepper in a big bowl.

- After stuffing the sausage mixture into each mushroom cap, arrange them on a baking sheet.
- Bake for 20 minutes in a preheated oven, or until golden brown and cooked through.

Cheese-Stuffed Meatballs

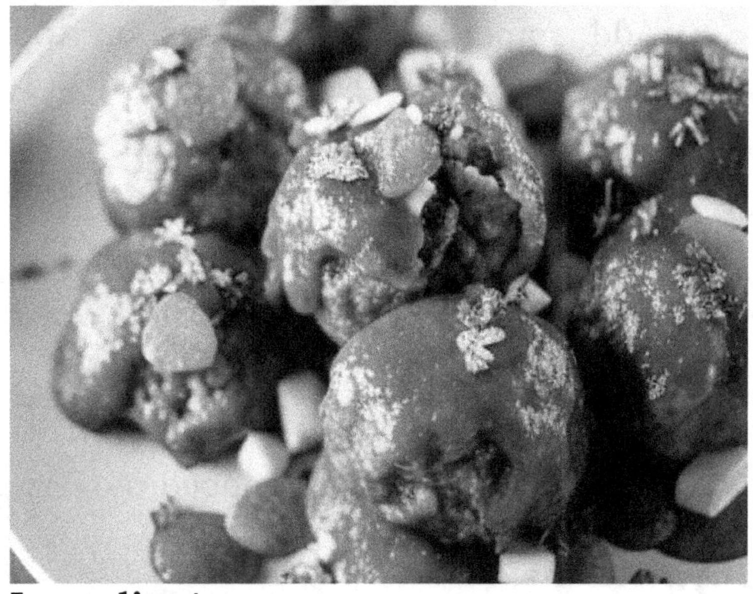

Ingredients:
- 1 pound of ground beef and 1/2 cup of breadcrumbs.
- 1/4 cup Parmesan cheese, grated - 2 minced garlic cloves
- 2 teaspoons freshly chopped parsley
- 1/2 cup of mozzarella cheese, shredded

- To taste, salt and pepper

Instructions:
- Set the oven to 375 degrees.
- Combine the breadcrumbs, Parmesan cheese, garlic, parsley, salt, and pepper in a sizable bowl with the ground meat.
- Create 12 equal pieces of the mixture into balls.
- Create a little divot in each meatball and insert a few mozzarella cheese slices.
- Arrange the meatballs on a baking sheet and bake for 20 minutes, or until fully cooked and browned.

Lamb Kebabs with Mint Sauce

Ingredients:
- 2 pounds of ground lamb;
- 1 cup of diced onion; and 2 minced garlic cloves.
- 2 teaspoons freshly chopped mint
- Olive oil, 2 tablespoons
- To taste, salt and pepper
- Garlic Sauce:
- Half a cup of Greek yogurt
- 2 teaspoons freshly chopped mint
- 1 minced garlic clove

- One teaspoon of honey
- To taste, salt and pepper

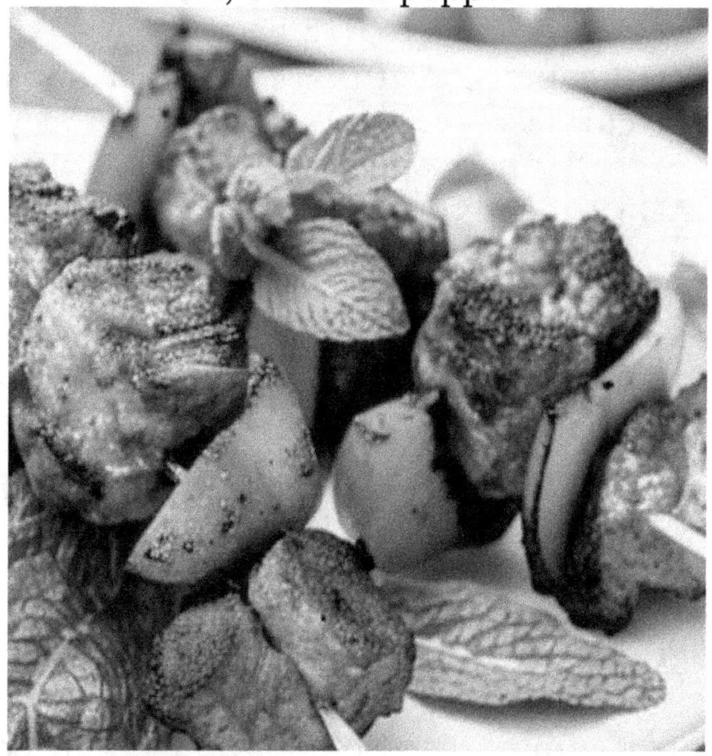

Instructions:

- Heat a grill pan or outdoor grill to a medium-high temperature.
- Combine the ground lamb, onion, garlic, mint, olive oil, salt, and pepper in a sizable bowl.
- Make 12 equal portions of the mixture into skewers by dividing it into equal portions.

- Cook the kebabs on the grill for 8 to 10 minutes, or until done.
- Make the mint sauce by combining the Greek yogurt, mint, garlic, honey, salt, and pepper in a bowl while the kebabs are cooking.
- Put the mint sauce on the side and serve the kebabs.

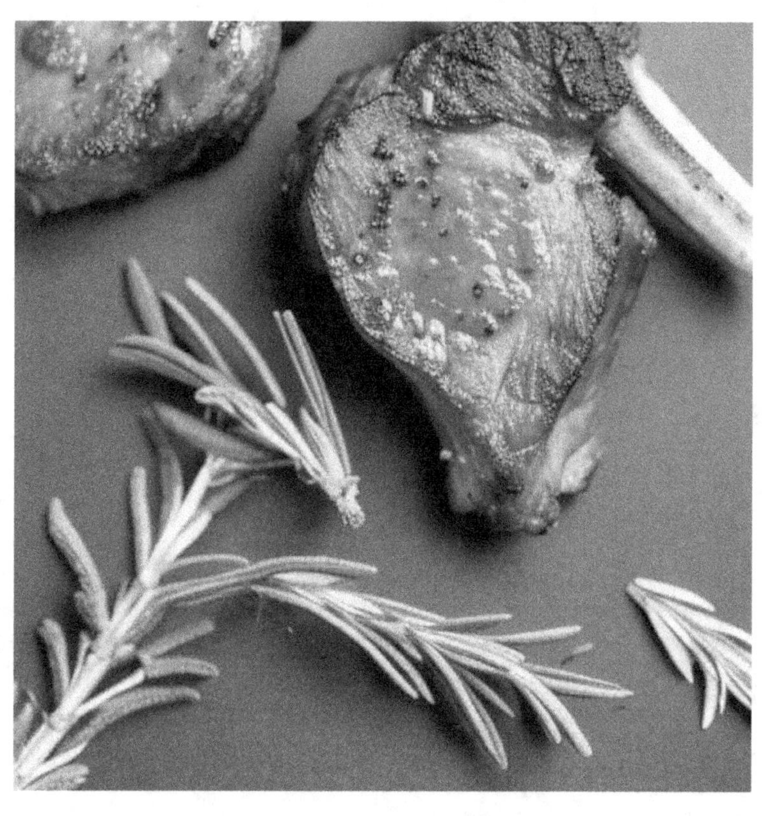

CHAPTER 5

SMOOTHIES RECIPES

Banana Protein Smoothie

Ingredients

- Bananas, one
- 1 serving of protein powder
- one cup of almond milk
- 1 teaspoon of honey
- 1 tablespoon of chia seeds

Strawberry Coconut Smoothie

Ingredients:

- Frozen strawberries, 1 cup
- 1/2 a banana
- half a cup of coconut milk
- 1-tbsp. honey and 1/2 cup ice

Blueberry Banana Smoothie

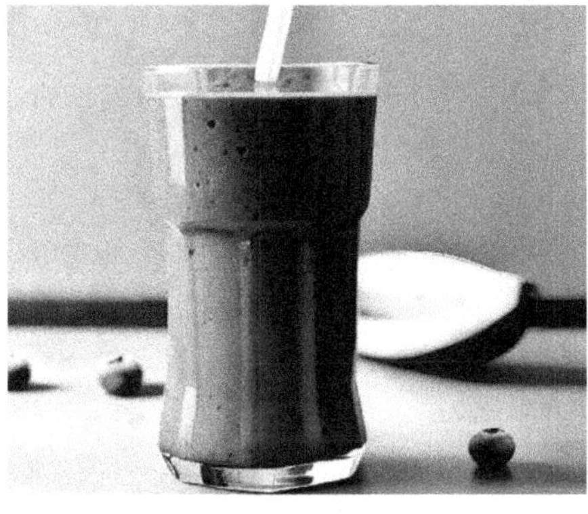

Ingredients:

- 1/2 a banana
- 1/2 cup blueberries, frozen
- half a cup of almond milk
- 1 teaspoon of honey
- 1-half cup ice

Tropical Smoothie

Ingredients:

- 1/2 a banana
- 1/2 cup pineapple chunks, frozen
- 1/2 cup mango chunks, frozen
- half a cup of coconut milk
- 1 teaspoon of honey
- 1-half cup ice

Instructions:

- put all the ingredients inside the blender
- Blend until creamy and smooth.
- Enjoy!

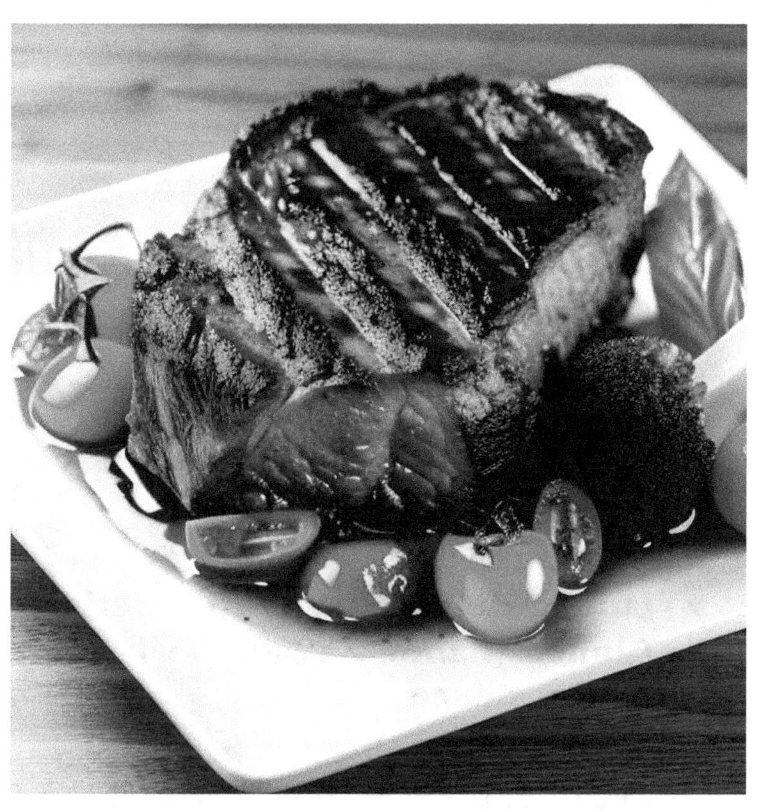

CHAPTER 6

MEAL PLAN

Day 1

- **Breakfast**: Bacon and eggs
- **Lunch: Turkey Burger with Avocado**
- **Dinner:**
- **Cumin-Spiced Beef Ribs**

Day 2

- **Breakfast**: Sausage and eggs
- **Lunch: Keto-Friendly Beef Jerky:**
- **Dinner: Lamb Kebabs with Mint Yogurt Sauce**

Day 3

- **Breakfast: Pancakes with bacon and eggs**
- **Lunch: Beef and Broccoli Stir Fry:**
- **Dinner: Grilled Beef Steak:**

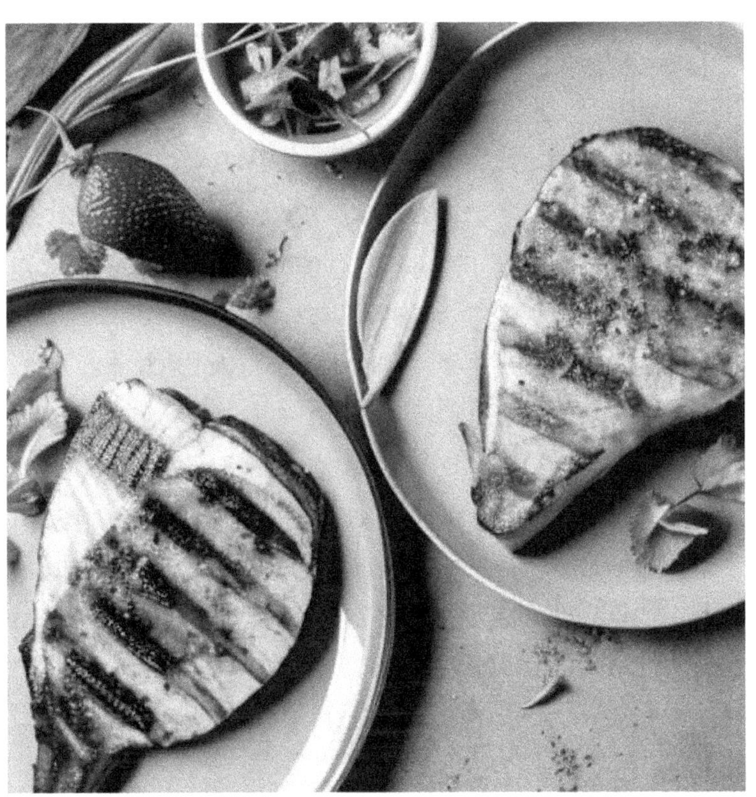

CONCLUSION

In general, the carnivore diet is an effective strategy for women who want to reduce their weight and get better health. Those who are ready to give it a go could be pleasantly pleased by the outcomes, even if it might not be for everyone. You may have the body and energy levels of your dreams by adhering to a few straightforward rules and including lots of nutritious animal products in your diet. Why not thus try the carnivore diet and see what results it has for you? With you may succeed on this unusual and fruitful diet.

I'm grateful that you took the time to read my book. I hope you like it and it gave you something to think about. Thank You

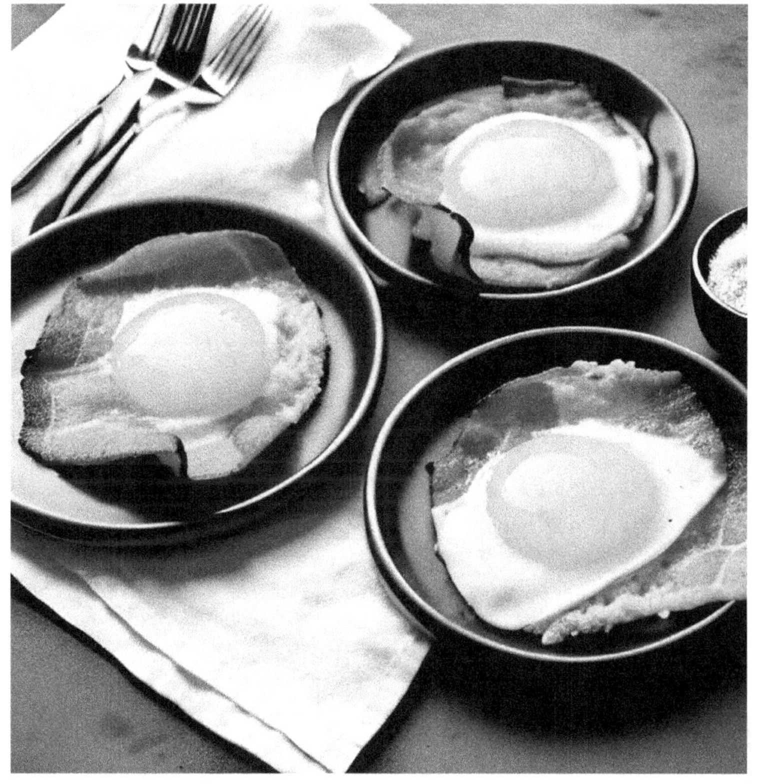

DAILY MEAL PLANNER

TO DO		EXERCISE
1		
2		
3		**GOAL ACTIVITIES**
4		☐
5		☐
6		☐
7		☐
8		☐
9		☐
10		☐

SHOPPING

<table>
<tr><td colspan="2" align="center">MEALS</td></tr>
<tr><td>BREAKFAST</td><td></td></tr>
<tr><td>LUNCH</td><td></td></tr>
<tr><td>DINNER</td><td></td></tr>
<tr><td>SNACKS</td><td></td></tr>
<tr><td>DESSERTS</td><td></td></tr>
</table>

INSPIRATION

NOTES & TIPS

DAILY MEAL PLANNER

TO DO

1	
2	
3	
4	
5	
6	
7	
8	
9	
10	

EXERCISE

GOAL ACTIVITIES

	☐
	☐
	☐
	☐
	☐
	☐
	☐

SHOPPING

<table>
<tr><td colspan="2" align="center">MEALS</td></tr>
<tr><td>BREAKFAST</td><td></td></tr>
<tr><td>LUNCH</td><td></td></tr>
<tr><td>DINNER</td><td></td></tr>
<tr><td>SNACKS</td><td></td></tr>
<tr><td>DESSERTS</td><td></td></tr>
</table>

INSPIRATION

NOTES & TIPS

DAILY MEAL PLANNER

TO DO	
1	
2	
3	
4	
5	
6	
7	
8	
9	
10	

EXERCISE

GOAL ACTIVITIES

	☐
	☐
	☐
	☐
	☐
	☐
	☐

SHOPPING

<table>
<tr><td colspan="2">MEALS</td></tr>
<tr><td>BREAKFAST</td><td></td></tr>
<tr><td>LUNCH</td><td></td></tr>
<tr><td>DINNER</td><td></td></tr>
<tr><td>SNACKS</td><td></td></tr>
<tr><td>DESSERTS</td><td></td></tr>
</table>

INSPIRATION

NOTES & TIPS

DAILY MEAL PLANNER

TO DO	
1	
2	
3	
4	
5	
6	
7	
8	
9	
10	

EXERCISE

GOAL ACTIVITIES

- ☐
- ☐
- ☐
- ☐
- ☐
- ☐
- ☐

SHOPPING

<table>
<tr><td colspan="2">MEALS</td></tr>
<tr><td>BREAKFAST</td><td></td></tr>
<tr><td>LUNCH</td><td></td></tr>
<tr><td>DINNER</td><td></td></tr>
<tr><td>SNACKS</td><td></td></tr>
<tr><td>DESSERTS</td><td></td></tr>
</table>

INSPIRATION

NOTES & TIPS

DAILY MEAL PLANNER

TO DO	
1	
2	
3	
4	
5	
6	
7	
8	
9	
10	

EXERCISE

GOAL ACTIVITIES

- ☐
- ☐
- ☐
- ☐
- ☐
- ☐
- ☐

SHOPPING

<table>
<tr><td colspan="2" align="center">MEALS</td></tr>
<tr><td>BREAKFAST</td><td></td></tr>
<tr><td>LUNCH</td><td></td></tr>
<tr><td>DINNER</td><td></td></tr>
<tr><td>SNACKS</td><td></td></tr>
<tr><td>DESSERTS</td><td></td></tr>
</table>

INSPIRATION

NOTES & TIPS

DAILY MEAL PLANNER

TO DO

1	
2	
3	
4	
5	
6	
7	
8	
9	
10	

EXERCISE

GOAL ACTIVITIES

- ☐
- ☐
- ☐
- ☐
- ☐
- ☐
- ☐

SHOPPING

MEALS

BREAKFAST	
LUNCH	
DINNER	
SNACKS	
DESSERTS	

INSPIRATION

NOTES & TIPS

DAILY MEAL PLANNER

TO DO	
1	
2	
3	
4	
5	
6	
7	
8	
9	
10	

EXERCISE

GOAL ACTIVITIES

- ☐
- ☐
- ☐
- ☐
- ☐
- ☐
- ☐

SHOPPING

MEALS	
BREAKFAST	
LUNCH	
DINNER	
SNACKS	
DESSERTS	

INSPIRATION

NOTES & TIPS

DAILY MEAL PLANNER

TO DO	
1	
2	
3	
4	
5	
6	
7	
8	
9	
10	

EXERCISE

GOAL ACTIVITIES

	☐
	☐
	☐
	☐
	☐
	☐
	☐

SHOPPING

<table>
<tr><td colspan="2">MEALS</td></tr>
<tr><td>BREAKFAST</td><td></td></tr>
<tr><td>LUNCH</td><td></td></tr>
<tr><td>DINNER</td><td></td></tr>
<tr><td>SNACKS</td><td></td></tr>
<tr><td>DESSERTS</td><td></td></tr>
</table>

INSPIRATION

NOTES & TIPS

DAILY MEAL PLANNER

TO DO

1	
2	
3	
4	
5	
6	
7	
8	
9	
10	

EXERCISE

GOAL ACTIVITIES

- ☐
- ☐
- ☐
- ☐
- ☐
- ☐
- ☐

SHOPPING

<table>
<tr><td colspan="2">## MEALS</td></tr>
<tr><td>**BREAKFAST**</td><td></td></tr>
<tr><td>**LUNCH**</td><td></td></tr>
<tr><td>**DINNER**</td><td></td></tr>
<tr><td>**SNACKS**</td><td></td></tr>
<tr><td>**DESSERTS**</td><td></td></tr>
</table>

INSPIRATION

NOTES & TIPS

DAILY MEAL PLANNER

TO DO	
1	
2	
3	
4	
5	
6	
7	
8	
9	
10	

EXERCISE

GOAL ACTIVITIES

☐
☐
☐
☐
☐
☐
☐

SHOPPING

MEALS	
BREAKFAST	
LUNCH	
DINNER	
SNACKS	
DESSERTS	

INSPIRATION

NOTES & TIPS